YOUR JOURNEY TO
CALM

A Guide to Leaving Anxiety
and Panic Attacks Behind

MAGGIE OAKES

♡AFFIRMATIONS FOR ANXIETY♡

As a thank you for buying my book I'm giving you an exclusive free video on affirmations for anxiety. Watch it daily for maximum effect.

Download the video here: https://gumroad.com/l/oBrDm

All of the downloadables can be found here: https://gumroad.com/calmwithmaggie

This book is dedicated to everyone
suffering from anxiety.

May you find peace

May you find happiness

May you be calm

The author of this book is a medical doctor doing her residency in psychiatry, but in order to protect the privacy of her patients and the author as a doctor this book is written under a pen-name.

CONTENTS

INTRODUCTION

In recent years the number of people suffering from mental health problems has risen alarmingly fast - with anxiety and panic attacks affecting as many as 3 in 10. Everybody feels anxiety at some point in their lives; starting a new job, moving home, sitting an exam, going on a first date, we expect to feel anxious and have butterflies in our stomachs. But for anyone suffering with anxiety or panic attacks such feelings are very much amplified, much more frequent (sometimes daily) and don't necessarily correspond to external events.

If you suffer from either anxiety disorder or panic attacks, or both, you have come to the right place. In this book I delve into the world of these disorders, looking at what may cause them and the various things you can do about them. From tips on self-help to information on professional help, from your feelings to the science behind them.

NOTE: *If you are suffering with a panic attack or acute anxiety right now and need fast relief,* *turn to Chapter 4, where you will find some tips on what you can do to help yourself.*

You may wonder what qualifies me to write this book. First and foremost I am a fellow sufferer, I struggled for countless years with anxiety disorder, and also suffered with panic attacks for about five months. Secondly, I am a medical doctor currently doing my residency in psychiatry. I work with people suffering with mental health problems and have helped many with their anxiety and panic attacks.

I wrote this book to help you on the road to freedom from anxiety and panic attacks. Depending on the severity of your disorder and the length of time you have suffered with it, your journey may be faster or slower than others. What matters most is starting and knowing there is an end in sight. This book will not tell you to "get over it" or "it's all in your head". I have been where you are at right now, and I know how to help you get out of there.

Thanks to the knowledge I have shared in this book I myself have had my life changed for the better. I have also seen and treated many people in all walks of life based on the techniques mentioned here.

My promise to you is that after absorbing my tips and implementing them (it is no good just reading them) you will feel hope, you will become more courageous, and you will begin your journey to your dreamed-of life - a life free from anxiety and panic attacks.

Before reading any further, take a small break here, close your eyes, and imagine what your dream life looks and - most importantly - what it feels like. How will it feel to wake every morning without anxiety and panic attacks - or the fear of more anxiety and panic attacks? How will it feel to be confident and relaxed? What would your day consist of? Perhaps going for a walk, working out, shopping, spending quality time with your loved ones? Think of your dream life and make it feel real, use all of your senses. What will you see, hear and feel? Will you see smiles on the faces of your loved ones? Will you feel relaxed as you go about your day? Will you hear people telling you how well you look?

In the coming chapters I will show you what works and how to keep living the life you deserve. What you'll get is a combination of friendly advice and simple scientific explanations.

If your everyday life is ruined by unpredictable panic attacks or constant anxiety, then don't wait another second. Don't be beaten down by something you can AND WILL overcome. This is the moment you've been waiting for. The rest of your life starts here. Start today, start now. You can do this! All you have to do is turn the page and begin to claim your life back, step by step, day by day.

Keep this book with you at all times, so if you ever feel yourself in need of some advice you can dip into it wherever you are. Sometimes just reminding yourself that you are on a journey to recovery is enough to help calm you. Chapter 4 has 'fast relief' tips for those moments when you need some help quickly.

CHAPTER 1

WHAT QUALIFIES ME?

There are two things that qualify me to write this book and give you this advice. The main one is that I myself have suffered from both anxiety and panic attacks, so I understand and empathize with your pain. I suffered with anxiety for years, without even knowing what it was for some of those years. I also suffered with terrible panic attacks for many months. Everything was fine and then the next minute I couldn't breathe, it felt like I was having a heart attack. I thought I was going to die. I feared going outside alone or even leaving my bed - I was feeling completely lost in life.

But now - when I am on the other side of this story - I am grateful for the anxieties I have had (I understand that probably sounds a bit strange to you right now). I wouldn't be the strong person I am today without going through what I did. A dear friend once said to me: "Your soul was trusted to have this journey. You just need to realize why. What is the purpose?" I understand it now. I need to help people who are in that same dark place I was, I want to walk beside you on your journey and guide you to freedom.

The second thing that qualifies me, is that I am a medical doctor and I'm currently doing my residency in psychiatry. The human brain and it's secrets have long fascinated me.

One thing that has really sparked my interest in our brains is the placebo effect. A placebo is an inactive treatment or substance, such as a sugar pill or pretend procedure, that looks and feels just like a regular medical treatment. Studies have shown that if you think you're receiving a treatment, and you expect that treatment to work, it often does. To take things even further they have tried out placebo surgeries! One example is when a person needs knee surgery to relieve pain. They are put under general anesthesia and some small cuts are made into the skin around the knee, but nothing more. When the person wakes up their pain can be more manageable or even totally gone.

Just think about it - if we truly believe in healing then we can heal. The power of our mind is astounding.

I once had a young woman as a patient, who had suffered from social anxiety for about six years. She had gotten so accustomed to her anxiety she had forgotten what her life used to be like before it. Her anxiety had escalated so much she could barely leave her home to go to work. Her quality of life had deteriorated to such an extent that she finally decided to seek help. And help she got. With a combination of psychotherapy, counseling and antidepressants, she got back on her feet. Today she continues to get psychotherapy to keep her on track, but other than that, she is maintaining her good mental health on her own with different self-help techniques. She was really happy to have found the strength and courage to seek help - and stick at it.

That in the end is what determines our outcome - our willingness to seek help, and our persistence to stick at it. I hope you are in that place right now, to start changing your life and to put your trust in yourself and me. I cannot promise it will be easy, but it will definitely be worth it.

CHAPTER 2

SYMPTOMS AND THEIR CAUSES

Diagnosing and symptoms

In modern psychiatry, mental health disorders are defined using the classification from the Diagnostic and Statistical Manual of Mental Disorders (DSM for short). In short, the DSM is a manual that is published by the American Psychiatric Association to help mental health professionals diagnose their patients.

It might help to look at these explanations to get a better understanding of your own inner world. Of course not everyone has to be put into a certain box. What really matters is that you get the correct help.

Based on the DSM , anxiety disorders are divided into separate subcategories:

- generalized anxiety disorder

- panic disorder

- social anxiety disorder

- specific phobias

- obsessive-compulsive disorder

- post-traumatic stress disorder

- acute stress disorder

The techniques taught in this book are helpful with all of the subcategories, but I will go through the first three in more detail.

1. Generalized anxiety disorder (GAD)

According to the DSM, the person suffering from GAD has excessive anxiety and worry about some activities or events. As with most diagnoses there is also a time frame that has to be considered. To properly diagnose GAD the person has to have had these symptoms for at least 6 months, occurring on more days than not. This over-excessive worry makes it difficult living a normal everyday life and the person can't control the worry.

Although every person experiences GAD differently, some of the most common symptoms are:

- Palpitations, accelerated heart rate, shaking, sweating, dry mouth

- Difficulty breathing, feeling of choking, chest pain or discomfort, nausea

- Feeling dizzy or lightheaded, fear of losing control, fear of dying, feeling that objects are not real or that one's self is distant

- Hot flushes, cold chills, numbness or tingling sensations

- Muscle tension, inability to relax, feeling on edge, difficulty swallowing

- Difficulty concentrating, irritability, difficulty falling asleep

GAD is not caused by contact with a substance (for example drug abuse). Although alcohol, cannabis and even coffee may induce anxiety, this is not considered to be a type of anxiety disorder, because that person won't have symptoms of anxiety when they don't use these substances.

2. Panic disorder

This diagnosis is made when someone has recurrent unexpected panic attacks for at least one month and at least one of these symptoms: persistent concern about having panic attacks; worry about the implications or consequences of that attack (either losing control, going crazy, having a heart attack etc.); a significant change in behaviour because of these attacks.

People with panic disorder can also have social anxiety disorder. As with GAD, panic disorder is not caused by any substance abuse.

Panic attacks begin unexpectedly and they are an episode of intense fear. Usually during the attack the height of the fear reaches its maximum within a few minutes and lasts about 30 minutes - for some people even longer. Don't be alarmed if your panic attacks last for hours, what you're experiencing is one panic attack after another, there really is no time limit to them.

The symptoms of panic disorder are similar to those of generalized anxiety disorder, but the main things that sets them apart is that panic attacks are unpredictable and the person lives in fear of these attacks occurring again. Panic attacks are usually more intense and whilst panic attacks come and go, generalized anxiety disorder (as stated in its name) is generalized - the person suffers from it during most of the day.

3. Social anxiety disorder (agoraphobia)

A person suffering from this disorder has a persistent fear of one or more social situations where they are exposed to strangers or possible scrutiny by others. That person fears that he or she will do something embarrassing. Exposure to these types of situations provokes anxiety or even a panic attack.

Although the person knows that this kind of fear is unreasonable they still avoid all kinds of situations that might make them anxious. This interferes with their normal routine and functioning. And if they are in these situations, then they feel intense anxiety and distress.

In addition the person has these symptoms: blushing, fear of vomiting, urgency or fear of urination or defecation. In this case the symptoms are felt in the feared situations only - for example speaking or eating in public, being at parties, meetings or classrooms.

Like the previous disorders - social anxiety disorder is not caused by substance abuse.

Why is this book concentrating on these three subcategories? Because I have experienced them all and have found that their therapeutic approach is similar.

It is also worth mentioning that many times these conditions overlap and one can turn into the other. When people experience panic attacks they may be afraid to go to work or even to go outside. But avoidance will make the fear even stronger. This can escalate to the sufferer being frightened all day long and experiencing symptoms of generalized anxiety.

Simplified science behind the symptoms

The brain contains about 100 billion nerve cells called neurons whose function it is to process and transmit information. In order for our brain to do its job the neurons must communicate with each other. Information is exchanged between them via chemicals called neurotransmitters, which send information from one part of the brain to another. In a healthy person's brain everything is balanced - the neurons are working correctly and the neurotransmitters are secreted in the right amounts.

The main neurotransmitters in the brain related to symptoms of anxiety are serotonin, dopamine, noradrenaline (norepinephrine) and GABA (gamma-aminobutyric acid). Each of them affects the neurons differently through their own receptors - small seats on the neuron walls, where the neurotransmitters bind to the neuron. By taking a seat there, the neurotransmitters can have their effect on the neurons. To take this even further, there are very many types of receptors and the activation of some leads to tranquilizing effects while the activation of others might lead to symptoms of anxiety. It's a complicated system.

In the case of anxiety disorders and even depression these "conversations" between the transmitter and the neuron are defective. It really depends on the person and disorder, but in many studies it is shown that people with anxiety have less serotonin than those without anxiety. Serotonin is usually associated with relaxation and happiness. In some people the problem might be that they don't produce enough serotonin, whilst in others there might not be enough serotonin receptors. These people need different approaches to their treatment - so when choosing the right medication, it is important to know which receptors to activate and which to de-activate. I must reiterate that everyone is different and this is why certain medications work for some people and not for others.

A small pea-sized part of the brain, called the pituitary gland, secretes a transmitter named corticotropin in response to stress, it then travels through the body and stimulates the adrenal gland to produce cortisol - better known as the stress hormone. Some of cortisol's effects include weakening your immune system, reducing bone formation, lengthening wound-healing time, and activating anti-inflammatory pathways. It also makes large amounts of blood sugar available for energetic purposes, which has evolutionary been important for the fight-or-flight response. When something unexpected happens (for example something frightening) this circuit is put into action and we have a surge of cortisol flowing in our blood.

This is why in some cases the disorder can't be defeated by just meditating or working-out. The chemical imbalance (that may have occurred and built up for some years) might need to be corrected with the help of certain types of medications. So in more difficult cases the combination of both self-help and professional help yields the best results - more on that in Chapters 5 and 6.

What causes these disorders?

The short answer is, it's a combination of genetics and environment. But let's look at these two factors in more detail.

If a person has gone through a lot of trauma early-on in their life, then these events shape the way neurons develop and communicate with each other in their brain, possibly leaving that person more vulnerable to stress. You might say that fear becomes encoded in their mind.

For example, social anxiety can be caused by low self-esteem, which could have been triggered by an experience such as being laughed at in a classroom after answering a question incorrectly. Panic attacks might be triggered by different events - illness, accidents, loss of someone close to you or other traumatic experiences. Someone who has already experienced panic attacks before will have a heightened sensitivity to the elevation of their heart rate, making it easier for them to experience another panic attack.

There have been a wide variety of research studies into the genetics of anxiety disorders, many of which have found that if a person's close relative has any sort of mental illness then that person themselves is predisposed to getting the same illness. But actually getting that same disorder is more complicated, which is where environmental factors come into play. Let's say, for example, you have the genes for developing social anxiety, but you are brought up in a loving family, your efforts are always supported and you socialize with a lot of nice people, then you probably are confident and the likelihood of you getting social anxiety is far smaller. At least smaller when compared to someone with similar genes who has had a more difficult upbringing. So again, mental health problems are really complicated and it is difficult to say which one thing caused them.

What else might cause symptoms of anxiety and panic attacks?

Sometimes other medical conditions or substances can cause anxiety - for instance, as mentioned before, anxiety can be induced by certain types of drugs, alcohol and caffeine. If you think drugs, alcohol or caffeine may be causing your problems, then seek help if you cannot just cut them out yourself. Medical

Doctors look at the spectrum of possible reasons for symptoms - ranging from the simplest and least problematic to the most severe and life-threatening. The doctor bases the differential diagnosis on his experience observing these symptoms, their frequency, location, and severity, as well as the patient's medical history. A thorough check up with your doctor is recommended to ensure there is no underlying medical cause for your symptoms.

Let's have a look at a few medical conditions that can cause anxiety symptoms.

Hyperthyroidism

The pituitary gland secretes a plethora of transmitters into the bloodstream - one of them is thyroid stimulating hormone (TSH), which stimulates the release of thyroid hormones from the thyroid. If the production of TSH is in overdrive then it means that more and more thyroid hormones are produced. This condition is called hyperthyroidism. It's symptoms include increased sweating, fast heart rate, weight loss, nervousness, and difficulty sleeping. All symptoms very similar to anxiety.

Hypercortisolism

Previously in this chapter we talked about how our bodies produce cortisol. There are conditions where the production of cortisol is too high, making that person suffer from chronic stress. So here the symptoms may present like anxiety, but the problem is a medical one.

Unhealthy digestive tract

The number of scientific research studies into the connection between gut microbes and mental health issues is on the rise. I myself have read through many of these research papers and based on their findings and my own experience can conclude that in some cases anxiety is caused by problems in our digestive tract.

For example, for people with either gluten intolerance or sensitivity, gluten destroys (to varying degrees) the normal architecture of the walls in their small intestine, thus letting in harmful bacterial toxins from the digestive tract. The theory here is that these toxins affect different systems in the body, leading to stress or anxiety. Gluten sensitivity is also characterized by digestive issues, fatigue and headaches. Some people with gluten sensitivity have symptoms that are so mild they never get diagnosed.

This doesn't mean to say that everyone who is suffering from anxiety should go on a gluten free diet, but there is no harm in cutting out gluten for 3-4 months and seeing if your anxiety gets better during that time

Always seek a doctors help in either outruling or discovering other conditions that may be causing your anxiety or panic attacks, but do some of your own detective work too. Ask yourself:

What is my backstory?

Has there been anything in my past that might have predisposed me to having this disorder?

When and how did the symptoms start, and how have they changed over time?

Have I been drinking too much alcohol or using any drugs?

Am I getting enough sleep?

Do I have any symptoms that don't correlate with anxiety or panic attacks?

The answers to these questions will help you - and your doctor.

CHAPTER 3

SETTING YOURSELF UP FOR SUCCESS

Before we deal with your anxiety there are a few things to do that will set you up on your quest for success. It's important to trust in yourself; to trust in your ability to do all that is necessary to get better. If you are in any way doubting your ability to take this journey, know that there are many who have been in a similar position to you who are now living anxiety and panic free - me included! If they can do it - SO CAN YOU.

Firstly, you can make your journey through this much easier by approaching it with a positive mindset. Be kind to yourself and believe that your life will take a turn for the better.

Here are a couple of exercises to help. These will be much more effective if you relax before doing them - sit comfortably, close your eyes, take a few deep breaths and relax your muscles. I suggest you try both of these exercises:

1. Imagine yourself in a situation where you have recently been overly anxious. Now take a minute and imagine yourself back in that situation but this time in a calm frame of mind. See yourself calm and in control, feel yourself relaxed and at ease. Would you be happier? Would you do anything differently in that situation if you didn't have anxiety? Take your time and use all of your senses to imagine this scenario. How much better will your life be when you can approach life in this calm way?

2. Imagine the things you would do if you didn't have anxiety or panic attacks. Take a while to think about this, because this will be your motivation. It doesn't have to be anything monumental. It could just be walking in the park or getting your groceries. Maybe going to the movies, hanging out with your friends, travelling to the city you've always dreamed of. My motivation was just to feel safe being alone and not having my phone with me - as simple as that. It can really help if you know why you are doing this and why you want to get better.

Now you have found your motivation, write it down, draw it or make a collage of pictures from magazines to illustrate it - a sort of a vision board for living a life free from anxiety and panic.

Make a list of things you really want to do, for example :

When my life is anxiety-free I will ...

Drive my car

Go to the grocery store

Sit and enjoy a nice warm croissant in a cafe

Go backpacking

etc.

Put this motivating list somewhere you can regularly see it - either on your wall, by your bed, on your desk or in your wallet, whatever suits you best (you could have one copy for at home and one that you carry around with you) . This will be your anchor, your vision for a brighter future. If ever the going gets tough, a look at this can be your motivation to keep on moving towards the future you dream of.

The next step is to encourage yourself. I recommend you stand in front of a mirror, relax your shoulders, take a couple of deep breaths, look deep into your eyes and smile. Say to yourself in the mirror: "I can do this. I will get better. I am not alone". Say it a few times -

and feel it. You could also adopt the Superman pose - hands on your hips, straighten your back, hold your head up high and feel your inner strength. The very fact that you are reading this book proves that you have taken the first courageous step towards your freedom. I believe in you.

If you have not yet told anyone else about your anxiety or panic attacks, then now is the time to consider opening up to someone. Either join a support group or see a professional. People often find relief when they talk to someone. I didn't tell anyone about the magnitude of my panic attacks for a long time, but when I did open up, I felt stronger for doing so.

A good idea is to score yourself when starting on your journey of healing, then score again later to track improvements. Score yourself on a scale from 1-10 below. You'll want some of these scores to go up and others to go down:

- How well do you sleep?

- Do you exercise regularly?

- Do you drink plenty of water every day?

- How healthy is your diet?

- How much does your anxiety/panic attacks rule your life?

- How bad is your anxiety?

- Do you feel hopeful of your life getting better?

CHAPTER 4

FAST RELIEF

This chapter is for those who are having an anxiety or panic attack *right now* and need quick results (see Chapter 5 for help for long-term results) .

What are you struggling with at this moment? An acute panic attack? Anticipation anxiety? Social anxiety? Pick a scenario you feel describes you best at this very moment and go to the appropriate section below. If you feel none of these apply to you 100%, then choose the panic attack option - the suggestions listed there are useful for all types of anxieties.

Panic attack

Does your world feels like it's caving in and smothering you? I know this won't make it any easier, but trust me when I say that this will pass and it won't kill you. Breathe calmly and release any tension in your body. Yes, you may feel dizzy or on the verge of a heart attack, but that is the adrenaline coursing around inside of you. Adrenaline causes high blood pressure, increased heart rate and rapid, shallow breathing. You will sweat more because of the adrenaline, your mouth will be dry, and you might feel tingling in different parts of your body. These are all normal elements of an anxiety or panic attack.

What is your worst case scenario currently? Probably that you are going to die or embarrass yourself in some way. As I said before, you are not going to die of this panic attack - it will pass and you will be fine. You have come through them before and you will come through this one. And it is also unlikely that you are going to embarrass yourself - people take less notice of us than we think at times and you do not have a big red sign on your forehead flashing 'PANIC'. And if you do need to turn to someone for some support, you may also be surprised by how compassionate and caring people can be (and how many of them will suffer/have suffered/know someone who suffers with anxiety and panic).

Even though you may feel like this panic attack will never go away, the truth is that panic attacks usually last up to 30 minutes, in some cases they go away faster, in some cases slower. You have made it this far - well done.

One of my favourite self-help techniques is to use all of my senses, one by one. Go through these prompts slowly, really concentrating on each one:

- Let's start with **Sight** - stay wherever you are and slowly look around you. What things can you see? What colours are there? Can you see your favourite colour? Is there any movement? What is your favourite thing you can see?

- **Sound** - you can close your eyes for this, if it feels better. What can you hear? Can you isolate the sounds? Where are they coming from? What/who is making those sounds? How many sounds can you hear? Is there a favourite?

- **Smell** - what can you smell? How would you describe it? Where is it coming from? Are there any scents you particularly like?

- **Touch** - are you sitting down or are you standing up? What do you feel against your body? Hold something in your hand, feel the texture, feel the temperature, describe this object in your mind. Try this with different objects.

Are you feeling better now? If not go through the above exercise again - seeking different sensations. Or read through the next sections for anxiety in case there is something in there that will help you. Some people find counting backwards from 100 helps - another option is to think of an item for each number, so 100 balloons, 99 lollipops, 98 flowers, 97 cars, 96 puppies, and so on.

Anticipation anxiety

When you're feeling anxious about possibly feeling anxious, your mind might be racing and thinking "hmm, maybe I don't need to go this appointment" or "I could always do that later". When this kind of thinking happens, realize that this is the fear talking. Challenge that fear. You might be imagining a frightful outcome to an upcoming situation, to combat this, think of a better outcome - think about yourself winning over anxiety, think about getting stronger with every step you take. Think about waking up tomorrow (or the day after whenever the event is) and knowing you DID IT - you survived and all went fine.

Maybe some forward planning will help? What can you do to prepare and make the event/day easier? Imagine where you're going and think if there is an easy way to escape from there - sometimes just having an escape route can make the situation more bearable, even if you're not going to use it.

Another support system can be a friend. Can you take a friend with you? Can you call a friend right now?

Promise yourself a reward afterwards. Perhaps something good to eat, a relaxing bath, a movie...whatever appeals to you. Think about that now and see how that changes how you feel.

Social anxiety

Know that getting better in the long-run means staying put right now, even if only for a short time - you CAN do it. Do your best to relax, allow your shoulders to drop and release any tension you feel in your body. Take a deep breath and let it out with a sigh. Know that this situation will not last forever.

If it makes you feel more comfortable, think of an escape plan from this situation. Just knowing you can leave at any time makes it more bearable. But don't escape just yet, have it as a back-up plan for now.

Concentrate on a sound, an object or even the texture of your own hand or clothes - whatever you can feel with your fingers. Focus on something that interests or comforts you - a flower, a picture, a view. You can also distract yourself by talking to someone friendly or concentrating on slowing your breathing. Check your posture, sit, stand or move like a confident person and look up and around. Smile. Changes in posture can make a difference to how we feel.

If you're feeling strong, then tell the anxiety to get even stronger. Challenge the anxiety. I have had help with thinking "come at me, show me what you got". Imagine yourself like a boxer in the ring, being bigger and stronger than the weakling boxer called anxiety. This may sound a little crazy when you are mid anxiety - but for some people it can really shift how they feel.

Stay in this situation as long as you can - every minute you stay is a victory and a step on the road to recovery. Try to stay in the social situation for just 5 or 10 minutes, making a promise to yourself that after that time you can leave. When the time is up, you might like to see if you can stay for even longer, or leave, both options are fine. Don't put yourself down if you can't make it that long.

My wish is that after following the suggestions above, you are now feeling a little - or a lot - better. We'll look at things to do for longer-lasting relief in the next chapter.

Do you have any other anxiety-relieving methods that have worked for you? Let me know at CalmWithMaggie@gmail.com

CHAPTER 5

SELF-HELP

If you have mild anxiety or panic attacks, then self-help techniques might be all you need. But I highly recommend you read the chapter 6 about professional help too - even just to broaden your views. I am a firm believer in combining lifestyle changes with different types of therapies and if really needed, medications.

What has definitely helped me the most is knowing the science behind anxiety and panic attacks and why running away from it only makes it worse. If we constantly avoid situations that make us anxious, then our brain is rewired to think that those situations actually are dangerous, thus causing the anxiety to grow even more. I often think (and sometimes say out loud): "Come at me! Show me what you got!" Now, you can't really yell it out in a grocery store, but you can muster up all your courage and yell it in your head. Don't fight anxiety, let it run its course.

Many people have found the following to be helpful:

Meditation

One of the first things people advise you to do when you suffer from anxiety is to start meditating and focusing on your breath. When you are really anxious, this is not going to work, in fact it could probably make it even worse for you. Someone who has anxiety is already too much concentrated on their bodily sensations.

For example, if you get anxious because of your heart beating faster and stronger, then when you try meditations which require you to concentrate on your breath or on your body, then inevitably you will become even more aware of your heartbeat and may spiral further into anxiety.

However, this doesn't mean that meditation doesn't work. It does! But you need to find a style that suits you and then practise it regularly. Maybe you could have a go at walking meditation - where you walk in a room or outside, and concentrate on different external senses; sounds, smells, the way your feet hit the ground.

If you feel more confident then surely try out breathing meditations as well, they are really effective when practised regularly. Meditation is great for the long term, it is something to start in your most relaxed moments, or when you are feeling better and then keep up as a kind of maintenance - as it is proven to reduce stress and anxiety when practiced for over three months.

Herbs

Different herbs can make you calmer. I really like different blends of natural herbal tea. A good way to de-stress is with a cup of tea. Some of the herbs that have extensive data to back up their calming effects are lavender, chamomile, green tea, lemon balm and ginger.

Sleep

It is very important to get enough sleep and improve your sleep hygiene. Most adults need 7 to 8 hours of sleep each night. Sleep is an important influencer in our mental health problems, yet it is often overlooked. I have seen so many people come to our clinic with different problems (depression, anxiety, manic disorder etc.) whose sleep cycles have drastically changed for one reason or another. Getting their sleep quality back in order has helped so many of them.

Take a look at your own bedtime routine. I recommend no phones and no screens for an hour before bedtime. During that hour do something quiet and calming. Slow down from the hectic day and allow yourself some me-time.

If you are in the habit of staying up late and would like to start going to bed earlier in order to get more sleep, it would be best to change the time you go to bed in small increments - for example start going to bed half an hour earlier each week, until you have reached your goal. Too big a change could be too much for your body clock.

Mindfulness

Start being more mindful in your life. Mindfulness means that the mind is fully attending to what's happening, to what you're doing, to what you are experiencing in the present moment. A great way to do this is to engage all of your senses one by one - what can you see, hear, smell, taste, touch right now? What textures can you feel right now? How do they feel? Are they warm or cold? Touch a surface with your hand - really look at it like a newborn child would. What sound does it make when you move your hand over it?

Try these types of exercises with different senses, let the world slow down and marvel at the things you normally don't pay attention to. Again, this exercise might be a bit scary to do when you're feeling anxious, but making a habit of being mindful really does make a difference. Every day when I walk to work I try being more mindful of my surroundings and it truly has made me calmer, because I used to spend my time on my walk thinking about the tasks I had to do.

Friends and family

Remind yourself that you are not alone on this journey. Our friends and family are here to support us. Some of them might have been through similar difficulties in their lives and might even provide you with useful tips. But I would suggest you also find some people who have not gone through the same things, because it can get tiring trying to get through your own fears and having to deal with someone else's too.

The internet is filled with people who have anxieties or panic attacks, there are many forums where we can share and learn from others - and sometimes it can be easier talking with a stranger through social media. It is good to share encouraging stories with each other.

Open up to someone, tell them you are struggling. For me it worked to let a friend know I got panic attacks when I went to the store, so when we went there together I automatically felt safer. I felt that I wasn't alone, that if I started feeling anxious, someone would assure me that I was strong enough. So please, let some of your closest friends and family know of your struggles.

Confidence

Fake it 'til you make it. No, don't fake that you don't have anxiety - for now it's a part of you and in time it will make you a lot stronger. One day you'll be happy you had anxiety or panic attacks, because in your struggles you will have learned and gained so much. By faking it, I mean act as if you feel confident - whether or not you are feeling anxious - by holding your head up high, straightening your back and feeling strong. Adopt the posture of a confident person. Straightening your back improves your breathing, which leads to less tensions and more oxygen for you.

I really enjoy standing in front of the mirror, making myself tall, straightening my body, putting my hands on my hips and smiling. I also imagine myself wearing a superhero cape that is moving epically in the wind - what a great way to start the day!

Self-help therapy

There are different types of therapies that are useful for anxiety disorders, for example CBT (cognitive-behavioural therapy) and behaviour therapy. Such therapies are best done by a trained therapist, but there are elements of these that can be done by yourself – as a self-help therapy.

A technique that has helped me a lot is self-awareness. Very simply this means being aware of your thinking and feeling. Research says we have up to 60,000 thoughts per day, with as many as 98 percent of them the same as we had the day before – so being aware of every single one may not be possible, but the more aware you can become of your thoughts the better. Be aware of your reactions to different situations and see what thinking pre-empted them. What are you saying to yourself in your mind? Talk kindly to yourself and be gentle with yourself. It's also important to recognize when you are overthinking or catastrophizing a situation.

A useful exercise is to list the situations/places that make you anxious – and then start to slowly go into these situations in a safe and controlled manner. When you plan ahead you can be prepared and give yourself the time you need, or even ask a friend to go along with you. For example, I was frightened of going to the grocery store and feared that I would faint in front of everybody. My first small step was to go to the store, but not go inside. The next step was to go and buy only one thing, so I knew I didn't have to spend a lot of time in the shop. Then day by day I took bigger steps and slowly got accustomed to the environment.

Write down your fears before going into the situation. What would be the worst outcome? And afterwards write down how you felt, what happened and what to do differently next time.

Doctor checkups

Fearing that you'll get a heart attack is a very common thought for people suffering with anxiety and panic attacks, and the more you focus on your fast beating heart, or the tightness in your chest, the worse the fear gets. It is a vicious cycle. This chapter is about self-help, but in that I would count 'helping yourself' by going and speaking to your doctor. There is nothing wrong with seeking reassurance by getting your blood analyzed, blood pressure checked or ECG done. Tell your GP what symptoms you are experiencing and let them know that it will really help if you could get your vitals and blood tests checked. Don't do this very often though - just do them once and reassure yourself that your heart is healthy. It can make all the difference to your recovery.

Practise different self-help techniques, do what you feel helps you the most in the moment . Keep practising and trust me, every small win will feel like heaven. And when you keep on getting better it's like a snowball effect; a small fearful human grows into a strong and confident superhero!

This chapter couldn't cover all the techniques available, but there are a few more examples in Chapter 7. If you have any other tips, anything that has worked for you and may work for another then please do let me know, I'm very keen to share as many self-help techniques with as many people as possible.

CHAPTER 6

PROFESSIONAL HELP

There is only so much we can do for ourselves. For some people their anxiety disorder, or any other medical condition for that matter, is mild and may not require professional help - or maybe only a small amount. But for some, their problems might be more difficult and require much more intervention. The best solution in my experience is to combine self-care, medications and therapy.

Two people can have a similar condition but it may be poles apart in terms of its severity. Let's look at an example to illustrate this: let's say Mary cuts her finger with some paper. Hurts right? But she doesn't even need a bandage or any painkillers, the cut is small and the pain dissolves on it's own. No professional help needed here. But what if Mary accidentally cuts off her finger? Herbs and meditation won't be of much help here. Yes, they can supplement the curative process, but Mary will clearly need much more professional intervention.

You might think that cutting off a finger is a bit too extreme of an example, but I think it gets the message across quite well. In both cases they were injuries to the finger and there was bleeding - but that's about as far as the similarities go. Anxiety and panic attacks can vary massively from one person to another, too.

If your anxieties have not faded in 3 months through using the self-care techniques I wrote about in the previous chapter, then it's likely that your disorder is not mild. It may be that the best approach for you would be to combine self-care with professional care.

Learn from my mistakes

Don't make the same mistake I did. I knew that antidepressants were used for panic attacks and anxieties, but I never thought that I would actually need them and left seeking help a little too long. When I started having my panic attacks I was still in medical-school. One thing we had (wrongly) been taught, was that we must never get ill. Our studies were so intensive that we daren't miss even a few seminars - if we did we sometimes had to repeat that subject because of those missed classes. So it became engraved in our minds that getting ill was *not an option*.

When I started having those panic attacks my first reaction was that I must be strong. So many thoughts ran through my head: "I'm a medical student, there is no way I can get ill", "I'm supposed to be healthy", "I'm supposed to be a role model", "I must be strong and carry on regardless". I thought that having panic attacks made me weak and unworthy of my profession. Oh, how wrong I was. Luckily I quickly realised my panic attacks were only getting worse and it was time to seek professional help.

Learn from me - there is nothing, I repeat *nothing* to be ashamed of. Not of your past, not of your experiences, not of your struggles and definitely not for seeking help. As a medical doctor, I can say that we are here to help people, that is why we became doctors, we thrive on helping others. We are not here to judge and we are also human - other doctors (like me) will have suffered with anxiety and panic attacks, too.

Where to begin?

Your GP (general practitioner) can prescribe psychiatric medications and most of them are qualified enough to start the treatment on their own, without you needing to see a specialist. Depending on where you're from, a GP might also be called a primary care physician.

Then there are different mental health professionals - psychiatrists, psychologists, counselors and nurses. Most people get them all mixed up, but the main differences are outlined here:

Psychiatrists are medical doctors, who have the license to prescribe medications. Some psychiatrists are also qualified to do therapies.

Psychologists deal with different types of counseling and psychotherapies - for example cognitive behavioral therapy, psychoanalytic therapy, music therapy, body awareness therapy etc. Psychologists have a doctoral degree in psychology.

Mental health counselors also provide counseling and psychotherapies. They have a master's degree in psychology.

Mental health nurses evaluate patients for mental illness and many of them are qualified to provide psychotherapy.

When comparing counseling and psychotherapy, the main difference is that counseling is for the short-term and deals with behaviour patterns. Whilst psychotherapy sessions last longer on the whole and focus on a wider range of issues.

With so many different professionals dealing with mental health, it can be overwhelming to know where to start from. One of the easiest ways is to consult with your GP or primary care physician first. Or you could make a phone call to a clinic that has different mental health professionals and ask them for guidance.

If you are already working with a mental health professional and don't feel like things are going as well as you would like, or maybe you feel you and they are just not a good 'fit', then it is most important to tell them so. Be honest. This is your health. Most of them understand that in order for the treatments to work you must get along with each other. If there is no trust or no connection, then it's more difficult to get good results. Ask them, maybe they can recommend someone who suits you better. Just don't lose hope, you'll find the right combination.

Antidepressants

Despite the name they are not just used for depression, some of them also work really well on anxiety disorders and panic attacks. They come under many different brand names - too many to list here. A few of the active ingredients in antidepressants that are helpful for anxieties are escitalopram, sertraline, paroxetine and tianeptine.

The main thing to remember with antidepressants is that they take time to work. You might be feeling small improvements in a few days, but the main effect comes after a few weeks of consistently taking them. That is why sometimes it is recommended to use an anxiolytic (anti anxiety drug) for the first few weeks that it takes the antidepressant to work. Oh, and for the medication to do it's magic, you need to take it as prescribed, which in most cases is every day, you won't see any feasible results if you aren't consistent in taking your medications.

Different people have different reactions to medications, so you might get different side-effects to someone else you know, or maybe even none. Even the medications themselves work differently in different people. One person might get better with small amounts of one drug whilst another needs another drug in higher doses. Again, don't lose hope if one medication doesn't work - there are other options to explore. It's important to know what medications you have tried, how long for and in what doses, so your doctor also knows what to try next. Keep track of when you are prescribed a medication, what it is, how long you take it for, the dosage - and how it works for you.

If you are on antidepressants and want to stop taking them, it is important that you come off them gradually and with help. Don't just suddenly stop one day - and don't quit on your own. Getting off medication can have nasty side-effects. The doses need to be slowly lowered for your organism to get used to being without the drugs. Seek your doctor's assistance in this.

Myths about antidepressants:

- Addiction - They are not addictive.

- Harmful - They are not poisonous, they are not made by huge corporate firms to make us all into zombies. Yes, there are some antidepressants that are not advisable to use when the person is pregnant or has cardiac problems, but all medications have some contraindications. And about feeling like a zombie? Some antidepressants do make people more dizzy, but those side-effects should go away in a few days. If not, then it is OK to consider using another antidepressant.

- Life-time treatment - In most of the cases you do not need to take antidepressants your whole life. The treatment usually lasts for about 6-12 months. In that time the chemicals in your brain get balanced out.

Anxiolytics

Anxiolytics are medications that inhibit anxiety. Other names for anxiolytics are tranquilizers and anti-anxiety medications. Some better known anxiolytics are alprazolam (e.g. Xanax), diazepam (e.g. Valium), lorazepam (e.g. Ativan) and clonazepam (e.g. Klonopin).

Usually I do not recommend the use of anxiolytics, because they are addictive and they only give a temporary relief. However, in some cases they are of great help. Earlier I mentioned that it takes time for antidepressants to start working and I feel that during that time it is helpful for some to use anxiolytics, as you don't need to use them for longer than a few weeks. In that time you do not get addicted to them. As with antidepressants, the doses need to be lowered slowly with guidance from your doctor.

I have had patients who didn't want to use anxiolytics and got by just fine before the antidepressants starting having their effect. It is an individual choice.

Other medications

There is one drug that isn't an anxiolytic, but in small doses it acts like one. It's called quetiapine. In high doses it is used in the treatment of different psychotic disorders. In medium doses it helps with depression. But in smaller doses, up to about 100mg a day, it aids with anxiety and sleep. It's not an anxiolytic and isn't addictive.

This is the drug that I have seen the best results with. However, its main side effects are dizziness and sleepiness (it is also used for sleep disorders), so it's not tolerated by many people. As with side-effects overall, the dizziness should subside in a few days.

What if my anxiety is caused by another disorder or disease?

If another disorder or disease is causing your anxiety then that needs addressing first. For example, people who have depression might also develop anxieties and once they recover from the depression it is most likely the anxiety will go away too. I wrote about some other medical conditions that cause symptoms of anxiety in Chapter 2.

I once heard an interesting analogy about depression, but I feel its meaning connects to anxiety disorders as well. Someone compared having depression to drowning in a glass of water: You are small and hopeless, stuck in a big glass filled with water. Medications can help you to rise to the top of the water, but you yourself have to make the effort of climbing out of the glass. I think this beautifully illustrates the importance of combining self-care with professional care.

CHAPTER 7

KEEPING THE BEAST DORMANT

Congratulations on getting to this point! You are feeling better now, more confident, more at ease. But don't get lazy, anxiety will try to creep back into your life when you least expect it. You have to change your lifestyle in order to stay calm and persevere.

Take my story for example. I suffered for years from anxiety disorder and when I got better I just took it for granted that all was well and life got back to 'normal' ; I felt healthy and thought that part of my life was behind me. It surely seemed that I had learned everything I needed from that experience. Nope it would seem not. After my panic attacks started I knew I had to actually change my way of life. I started meditating again, working out, being grateful and enjoying the small things in life. I put a small amount of time aside for myself every day, and a larger portion every week. I started making 'me' a priority. Follow my lead and start making 'you' a priority too.

How should you live your life in order to stay calm in the crazy world we live in?

Short answer - Do the things that you love to do.

Long answer - Same as the short answer, but in order to keep your body and mind in a state of tranquility you need to regularly practise different self-care techniques. You don't need to do all of these, just use the ones that work best for you.

Get out of your comfort zone

The number one thing that has helped me in the long run is doing the things that scare me. If my anxiety kept me from going to the stores, being physically active or socializing - then that is exactly what I kept on doing. If I needed to buy some groceries, I didn't talk myself out of it and say "Well, I don't actually need to buy those apples today, I can get them tomorrow". No, I just got out there and bought them. I highly suggest you keep on doing the things that you are/were frightened of the most. Scared of talking to strangers? Ask someone for directions on the street, or wish a cashier a lovely day. Afraid of being all alone in an unfamiliar place? Go and explore new places on your own. You probably know the things that scare you the most, don't try to cover them up - go and do them.

Meditation

Meditating is a good way to keep you calm. By making meditation a habit, we lower our stress levels and when something unexpected happens, we have a calmer reaction to it. Even overreacting to a positive surprise can put our minds into overdrive and cause an anxious reaction. There are many different types of meditation to choose from, I suggest you try as many as you can in order to find the one that suits you the best. I find guided meditations work best for me. I have struggled with meditating in silence and felt bad because I couldn't meditate "the real way". But here's the thing, there is no "real way". Meditation is meant to be helpful and whatever style you feel more comfortable with, that's the right meditation for you. The main thing is to feel good about what you're doing - then you will keep it up.

Workouts

Working-out is one of the most overlooked things regarding advancing our mental health. Yes, we might know that a healthy mind resides in a healthy body, but if you haven't experienced the positive emotions from working-out, then there's no real connection there for you. "Yes-yes, everyone says you should work out to be happier, but I don't feel a difference" - this was my mentality for years. If you're in the same boat that I was, then that most likely means that you haven't yet found your thing. Try out different trainings, give them a chance and if they are not for you then move on to the next one. Or maybe doing all kinds of varied workouts is your thing, with a new challenge every day. What I can tell you for sure is that working-out really does improve your mental health, it makes both you and your immune system stronger.

Be grateful

Keeping a gratitude journal is also helpful. I had a gratitude jar for a while - which meant writing down things I was grateful for on small pieces of paper, folding them and putting them in the jar. Then if I felt low I could take a few of the paper slips out and read them to remind me of all the positive things that had happened. This method didn't really work for me, because I wanted something I could take with me everywhere. What has worked for me, is writing three things I am grateful for each day in my gratitude journal - a small notebook I keep with me and can quickly open at any time to read something positive.

It is a great way to shift how I feel very quickly. I highly recommend it.

Writing your three things you are grateful for is best done before bedtime, because grateful thoughts can help you get a good night's sleep. I found it difficult at first to think of things to write down, but after some time it got a lot easier. You can write about how you had coffee with your friends, or saw a cat sunbathing. Be grateful for the simple things - having a roof over your head, a bed to sleep in and water on tap. Sometimes reminding ourselves of these blessings we take for granted can really shift how we feel. It is even more important to be grateful when it feels hard, because reaching for those good thoughts makes such a difference.

Now it is priceless for me to look back and see what I did on different days, for instance: *I am grateful that I watched an awesome movie with my family* - maybe not that big a thing to happen, but it brings back heartwarming memories.

Schedule self-care appointments

Keep track of your self-care routine. Have a journal where you plan out your week and set aside time for self-care. Even if planning is not your thing, I still suggest you make at least a note somewhere to remind you to take care of yourself, because during these busy times we often forget to carve out time for ourselves. A simple note beside your bathroom mirror reminding you to take a few deep breaths goes a long way.

Set aside some time for yourself and do the things you love. Now this is very different for everyone, but some of the most popular things to do are having a bath, taking a walk, being with a loved one, working on your hobbies, watching a movie, being outdoors, reading a book. You know yourself the best. Think about it for a minute, what actually makes you feel happy and relaxed? If possible take a whole day off a week just for yourself. But what might be even better, is to have 10-15 minutes of me-time every day.

Drink water

Drink plenty of water during the day. Being hydrated is a simple way of being healthy. When we don't get enough water our minds get foggy, it is difficult to concentrate and we might even get headaches. I keep a small bottle with me everywhere I go.

Another good tip is to drink a glass of water first thing after you wake up. The hours spent sleeping means your body is dehydrated. Drinking some water in the morning gets you up and going.

Healthy eating

Healthy eating is so important. There are many books, articles and blog posts on this subject. And so many diets to choose from. I would say that the more simple your diet, the better. For example, you should eat some fruits and vegetables daily, add less sugar to your food, eat less gluten and avoid junk food. That's it. And don't be too strict with your diet, because that will cause unnecessary stress.

The fresh fruits and vegetables give us important vitamins and minerals. Eating less sugar means a healthier liver and a healthier heart, among other benefits. Sugary foods can also make some people feel more anxious - so be aware of that. Gluten is found in different products containing wheat and rye and it can make some people feel foggy, bloated or even cause headaches. (More information about gluten sensitivity is in Chapter 2 under "Unhealthy digestive tract"). Try eating less gluten and see how it affects you. Junk foods have high levels of sugar and fat, so it's best to eat as little of them as possible. Look for healthier substitutes.

This doesn't mean you can't ever eat a piece of cake in your life. If you really fancy that cake, or that slice of pizza, then eat it and enjoy it. Getting a positive feeling from eating can make us happier and that's what our goal should be.

Sleep hygiene

Sleep, sleep, sleep. But not too much. You most likely know that getting enough sleep every day is monumental for your overall health. The cells in your body need that rest as much as you do. But oversleeping is just as bad for you as not getting enough sleep, it can leave you feeling groggy and unmotivated to do anything. It is ok to occasionally sleep longer when you haven't slept well for the last few days, or when you have strained yourself - both physically and mentally - but don't make it into a habit.

Affirmations

Affirmations are short, powerful statements. When you say them or think them repeatedly, they become the thoughts that create your reality because of their ability to rewire your brain. Much like exercise, they raise the level of feel-good hormones. Find affirmations that speak to you. Here are some examples:

I am good enough

I am creating a life that I love

I feel happy

I am loved

This is my time

I am feeling calm today

I am filled with gratitude

Write down different affirmations and speak them out loud. Which ones move you? Which ones motivate you? Try out different ones and really put some meaning into them. I like to say mine out loud in the morning.

Some say it takes 21 days of repetition for an affirmation to make its mark on your psyche, so aim to keep your affirmation going for at least a month. In the beginning you will have to consciously choose to repeat your affirmations. If you repeat them at every opportunity they will begin to replace the negative mind banter that takes over when we are not monitoring our thoughts.

Love yourself

Hug yourself when you wake up and say "I love you, I love you, I love you". Or say it while looking into your eyes in a mirror. Really mean it. Simple as that. This has done wonders for my self-esteem.

Mindfulness

Mindfulness means that the mind is fully attending to what's happening, to what you're doing, to what you are experiencing in the present moment. That might seem trivial, but we so often allow our minds to wander to replaying things from the past or worrying about things in the future - and that can make us anxious.

Practice mindfulness. Start out simple - for instance when you are eating focus fully on your meal, notice the taste and texture of the food, savour and enjoy every bite. Be mindful when you do a simple daily task like brushing your teeth *(OK, I confess I actually made notes for this bit of the book while brushing my teeth. Not very mindful I know, but I had to write these thoughts down before I forgot them.)* Being more mindful of things makes you notice and appreciate the small and awesome things in life.

Relationships

Communicate and socialize - either in person or over the internet if that suits you better. Facebook has lots of anxiety support-groups, you can find the most suitable one for yourself there. But of course a balance of both real life connections and internet friendships would be best.

There is also much evidence that being in a supportive community with good friends helps people live longer. Likewise loneliness does the opposite. So I encourage you to be with people in real life as much as possible, even if you're an introvert like me.

Being around like-minded people is good for you. Sharing stories, laughing, being there for each other - priceless. For me, there is nothing more gratifying than making another person smile.

No judgement

Practice being non-judgemental. Whether it is an emotion stirring up inside of you or someone driving their car too slowly in front of you. Don't judge, just experience the feelings. When I start getting an anxious reaction to something I feel the knot in my chest but I don't react to it in any way, I just let it be there, and the anxiety just disappears. When I see someone acting weird or honking their car horn at me, I do not judge them. They have their own life, their own feelings, their own experiences and reasons for doing things. It is never about me personally. I care about my health too much to let someone else's bad day influence my day.

Living in a non-judgemental way is so liberating, this has been one of the most important decisions I have made in my life. I am not perfect, from time to time I still judge others and myself, but what matters is that I notice that judgement and then change my way of thinking.

Do nothing

I took a week off from work recently and during that time I worked on personal development and my own projects. I was so productive and only did the things that I wanted, but even that wore me out after a while - constant to-do lists and goals can get tiring. So I took a day off from all the things I was doing, no more being productive, no tasks, just living and doing whatever I felt like for a whole day. A good portion of the day I spent eating good food and watching TV.

That was the most unproductive day I had, but I have no regrets, that was just what I needed. Less doing, more being.

Allow yourself to do nothing from time to time. Of course some of us thrive on being busy and if that is your jam, then you do it. Get to know what feeds you and do just that.

In this chapter we have looked at some of the ways you can keep your anxieties dormant or at least under control. There are many more and it is important to find what works for you. Earlier on in the book, in the section about medications, I said that for them to work you have to take them regularly. It's the same with self-care - for the best results do it regularly. Self-care should always be a priority - good health is a blessing that makes everything else in life so much easier. For these self-help techniques to really stick I suggest you keep track of them, mark out space in your diary - at least in the beginning before they have become a habit.

CHAPTER 8

HOW ARE YOU DOING?

When you have reached this point in the book I sincerely hope you are either better or well on your way there. I genuinely care. The main reason I wanted to become a medical doctor was because I thrive on helping others - friends and strangers alike. By now I hope that I am not a complete stranger to you anymore.

Check in with yourself:

- Am I feeling better? Slightly better or a lot better?

- What helped me the most?

- What helped me the least?

- What did I fear the most?

- What am I committed to continuing with?

- What tips did I ignore? Should I revisit those?

If you feel like sharing your journey, then please do so. You can contact me by my email or on my website (links are on the last page). Tell me what worked for you and what scared you the most. As I said before, I genuinely do care and I want to improve my knowledge on the subject in order to help even more people.

And as we did in chapter 3 - score yourself again from 1-10. Compare the results and see where you have improved - or where there is room for more improvement:

- How well do you sleep?

- Do you exercise regularly?

- Do you drink plenty of water every day?

- How healthy is your diet?

- How much does your anxiety/panic attacks rule your life?

- How bad is your anxiety?

- Do you feel hopeful of your life getting better?

What if I am not feeling any better?

Go through the tips in this book one more time and see if you really have done all you can do. This is a marathon not a sprint, you will have setbacks and change doesn't happen overnight. You need to believe in yourself and give it time. If that still doesn't help and you aren't doing so already, then I suggest you seek some professional help, from either a psychologist or a psychiatrist. If you already are getting professional help, then maybe you should find a new specialist, not everyone is specialized in anxiety or panic attacks. You should probably talk to them about it and ask if they can recommend someone more suitable for you. Also - do visit and talk with your doctor if nothing is improving.

ABOUT THE AUTHOR

Hi, I'm Maggie, your guide to a brighter future. Too cheesy? Well ok, maybe a little, but still truthful. I've lived a happy life - had a caring family, lived in a good neighborhood, obtained a great education, always had what I needed. But that still didn't protect me from the claws of anxiety. I suffered for years with social anxiety without even knowing what it was and not remembering that life used to be better. When I finally realized that I had anxiety I could not believe it. Were there really days in my past when I could freely go outside? I couldn't remember. Were there days I didn't have to worry so much? I honestly could not remember. But after years of suffering I got out of it, I could go wherever my heart lead me to. I was free.

Years later I had a health scare that caused me to have panic attacks mixed with generalized anxiety - but I got out of those as well. Now I am free again. I do my best to remember these experiences that have shaped me as a person.

I've always thrived on helping others, so I became a medical doctor. I pushed through medical school whilst having social anxiety, it was definitely not fun, but I made it - with great grades and heaps of knowledge. My path then led me to do my residency in psychiatry. I am fascinated by the intricate pathways in the brain and how they all connect and influence us.

I'm a friendly and (mostly) happy person, so throughout this book I wanted to add small smiley faces to brighten your day. That's how I usually write my e-mails, with happy emoticons. But it's not really conventional for a book to have smileys in it, is it? Well, this last page is about me, so here you go - have a smile and send one back to me :)

During my free time I like to spend time in nature. My biggest dream is to move to the countryside, help even more people and also have enough time for my hobbies. Some of my hobbies are hiking, yoga, nature photography and playing video games.

The contents of this book reflect my experience as a mental health sufferer and what I have been taught as a resident of psychiatry. The reason for writing this book is to help you. This is not solely based on my victory, it is also based on the journeys of the many people I have seen and helped.

THANK YOU FOR READING MY BOOK!

I really appreciate your feedback, and would love to hear what you have to say. Please leave me a helpful review on Amazon letting me know what you thought of the book.

Your input will help make the next version of this book and my future books better.

Thank You!

~ Maggie Oakes

Where to contact me?

E-mail: CalmWithMaggie@gmail.com

Links to all of my books, downloadables and the newsletter: https://linktr.ee/calmwithmaggie

Made in the USA
Middletown, DE
15 December 2019